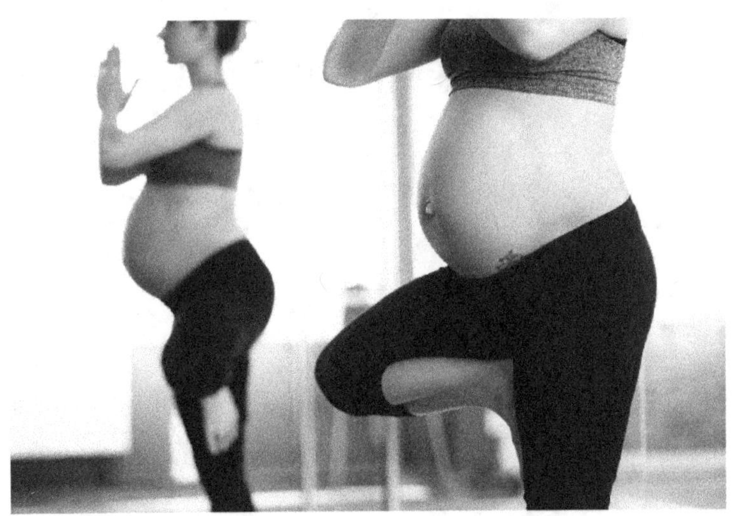

PREGNANT BUT FIT

A Guide to Fitness During Pregnancy

By Daniella Jabin

Copyright © 2023 by Daniella Jabin

TABLE OF CONTENTS

Introduction:

Embracing a fit pregnancy

Pregnancy is a transformative journey filled with joy, anticipation, and an overwhelming sense of responsibility. As an expectant mother, you are nurturing a new life within you, and it is only natural to prioritize your health and well-being throughout this incredible experience.

In the past, the prevailing belief was that pregnancy should be a time of rest and limited physical activity. However, recent research has shed new light on the benefits of exercise during pregnancy. It has become increasingly clear that staying active can have a positive impact on both the mother and the developing baby, leading to better overall health, improved mood, increased energy levels, and even shorter labor durations.

Welcome to "PREGNANT BUT FIT A Guide to Fitness During Pregnancy." This book is designed to be your comprehensive companion, offering guidance, insights, and practical advice on maintaining a fitness routine throughout your pregnancy journey. Our aim is to empower you with knowledge, debunk common myths, and provide safe and effective exercises tailored specifically for expectant mothers.

Authored by a team of experts in obstetrics, fitness, and nutrition, "PREGNANT BUT FIT" is a reliable and evidence-based resource that covers all aspects of prenatal fitness. Whether you are a fitness enthusiast or someone who is just beginning their fitness journey, this book will help you navigate the physical and emotional changes that come with pregnancy and enable you to make informed decisions about your health.

Inside these pages, you will find a wealth of information on the benefits of exercise during pregnancy, including its impact on cardiovascular health, muscular strength, and overall well-being. We will address common concerns and answer questions about exercise safety, modifying workouts for different stages of pregnancy, and dealing with discomfort.
However, this book goes beyond just exercise . We understand that pregnancy is a unique and personal experience, and we delve into the emotional and mental aspects of this transformative time. From managing stress and practicing self-care to embracing body changes and building a strong support network, we explore the holistic approach to well-being during pregnancy.

Our hope is that "PREGNANT BUT FIT" will not only equip you with the tools to stay active and healthy throughout your pregnancy but also inspire you to embrace this extraordinary journey with confidence and joy. With the right information and guidance, you can make pregnancy a time of empowerment, self-discovery, and celebration.

Let us embark on this remarkable adventure together, combining the love for your growing baby with the pursuit of a fit and healthy lifestyle. Get ready to nurture your body, mind, and soul as we dive into "PREGNANT BUT FIT : A Guide to Fitness During Pregnancy."

CHAPTER 1

UNDERSTANDING THE CHANGES IN YOUR BODY

Hormonal and physical changes

During pregnancy, a woman's body goes through numerous hormonal and physical changes to support the growth and development of the fetus. These changes are orchestrated by a complex interplay of hormones and are essential for a healthy pregnancy. Let's explore some of the key hormonal and physical changes that occur during this transformative period.

Hormonal Changes:

Human Chorionic Gonadotropin (hCG): The placenta produces hCG, which stimulates the ovaries to produce progesterone and estrogen. It helps maintain the uterine lining and supports the early stages of pregnancy.

Estrogen and Progesterone: These hormones play crucial roles in pregnancy. Estrogen helps stimulate blood flow to the uterus and breast tissue, while progesterone supports the growth of the placenta and helps maintain the uterine lining.

Relaxin: This hormone is responsible for relaxing the ligaments and joints in the pelvis, allowing for the expansion and flexibility needed during childbirth.

Oxytocin: Known as the "love hormone," oxytocin is responsible for stimulating uterine contractions during labor and helps with bonding between the mother and baby during breastfeeding.

Physical Changes:

Enlarged Uterus: As the pregnancy progresses, the uterus expands to accommodate the growing fetus. This can cause a visible bulge in the abdomen and a shift in the woman's center of gravity.

Breast Changes: The breasts undergo several changes to prepare for breastfeeding. They may become larger, tender, and more sensitive. The areolas (the dark skin surrounding the nipples) may also darken.

Weight Gain: Weight gain is a normal part of pregnancy, and it varies from woman to woman. The increased weight is due to the growing baby, amniotic fluid, placenta, and additional blood and fluid in the body.

Skin Changes: Many pregnant women experience changes in their skin, such as darkening of the skin in certain areas like the face (melasma), linea nigra (a dark line that forms on the abdomen), and stretch marks.

Increased Blood Volume: The body produces more blood during pregnancy to supply oxygen and nutrients to the growing fetus. This increase in blood volume can lead to changes in blood pressure and increased workload on the heart.

Digestive System Changes: Hormonal changes can affect the digestive system, leading to symptoms like nausea, vomiting (morning sickness), heartburn, and constipation.

Urinary System Changes: As the uterus expands, it puts pressure on the bladder, leading to increased frequency of urination. Hormonal changes also affect kidney function, resulting in increased urine production.

These hormonal and physical changes during pregnancy are natural and necessary for the well-being of both the mother and the developing baby. It is important for pregnant women to receive regular prenatal care to monitor these changes and ensure a healthy pregnancy.

skeletal and muscular adjustments

Pregnancy is a transformative period in a woman's life that brings about numerous physiological changes in her body. Alongside hormonal shifts and organ adaptations, the skeletal and muscular systems also undergo significant adjustments to accommodate the growing fetus and support the demands of pregnancy. This note explores the skeletal and muscular changes that occur during pregnancy and highlights their importance for maternal well-being and the development of the baby.

Skeletal Adjustments:

Postural Changes: As pregnancy progresses, a woman's center of gravity shifts due to the growing uterus. To maintain balance, the body compensates by altering the alignment of the spine, leading to changes in posture. The lower back curves inward (lordosis), the upper back becomes rounded, and the shoulders may roll forward.

Pelvic Changes: The female pelvis undergoes adaptations to facilitate childbirth. The hormone relaxin softens the ligaments and joints, particularly in the pelvic region. This increased flexibility allows the pelvic bones to widen, enabling the baby to pass through the birth canal during delivery.

Muscular Adjustments:

Abdominal Muscles: The rectus abdominis muscles (six-pack muscles) may separate along the linea alba to accommodate the expanding uterus. This condition, known as diastasis recti, is common during pregnancy and usually resolves postpartum with targeted exercises.

Pelvic Floor Muscles: These muscles play a crucial role in supporting the pelvic organs, maintaining continence, and assisting during childbirth. During pregnancy, hormonal changes and the weight of the growing baby place increased pressure on the pelvic floor, which can lead to weakened or stretched muscles. Engaging in pelvic floor exercises (Kegels) helps strengthen these muscles and minimize the risk of complications such as urinary incontinence.

Postural Muscles: The muscles of the back and hips, including the erector spinae, gluteal muscles, and hip flexors, may become strained due to the altered posture and increased weight during pregnancy. Gentle stretching and regular exercise targeting these muscle groups can help alleviate discomfort and maintain proper alignment.

Importance of Skeletal and Muscular Adjustments: The skeletal and muscular adjustments during pregnancy serve several essential purposes:

Support for the growing fetus: The skeletal changes, especially in the pelvis, allow for the baby's development and provide a pathway for childbirth.

Adaptation to the changing body: The adjustments in posture and muscle tone help accommodate the physical changes, reducing discomfort and facilitating day-to-day activities.

Preparation for labor and delivery: Strengthening the pelvic floor muscles and maintaining overall muscle tone can enhance a woman's ability to push during labor and aid in a smoother delivery process.

Pregnancy triggers significant skeletal and muscular adjustments to accommodate the growing fetus and support the physiological demands of pregnancy. Understanding these changes can help expectant mothers manage their well-being, engage in appropriate exercises, and seek necessary support during this transformative period. Maintaining a healthy skeletal and muscular system during pregnancy contributes to maternal comfort, facilitates childbirth, and promotes overall well-being for both mother and baby.

Cardiovascular and respiratory adaptations

Pregnancy is a remarkable physiological process that brings about numerous changes in a woman's body to support the growth and development of the fetus. Among these changes, cardiovascular and respiratory adaptations play a crucial role in ensuring an adequate oxygen supply and nutrient delivery to both the mother and the developing baby. This note aims to provide an overview of the key adaptations that occur in the cardiovascular and respiratory systems during pregnancy.

Cardiovascular Adaptations:

Increased Blood Volume: Pregnancy triggers a substantial increase in blood volume, which starts as early as the first trimester and continues to rise throughout pregnancy. This adaptation serves to meet the metabolic demands of the developing fetus and prepare for potential blood loss during childbirth.

Cardiac Output Enhancement: Cardiac output, the volume of blood pumped by the heart per minute, significantly increases during pregnancy. This increase is primarily attributed to a rise in stroke volume (the amount of blood pumped with each heartbeat) rather than an elevation in heart rate. Cardiac output can be up to 50% higher by the third trimester compared to pre-pregnancy levels.

Maternal Heart Rate: Resting heart rate slightly increases during pregnancy due to hormonal and physiological changes. It is common for heart rate to rise by around 10 to 15 beats per minute compared to pre-pregnancy values.

Blood Pressure Changes: Pregnancy induces changes in blood pressure regulation. During the first trimester, blood pressure may decrease slightly, reaching its lowest point around mid-pregnancy. However, as pregnancy progresses, blood pressure gradually returns to normal or slightly elevated levels by the third trimester.

Respiratory Adaptations:

Increased Oxygen Demand: The growing fetus requires an adequate oxygen supply, leading to an increase in the mother's oxygen consumption. This higher demand is met through adjustments in the respiratory system.

Altered Breathing Pattern: As pregnancy progresses, the diaphragm elevates due to the expansion of the uterus. This alteration in the position of the diaphragm results in changes to the breathing pattern, with an increased reliance on the expansion of the rib cage rather than the movement of the diaphragm.

Increased Minute Ventilation: Minute ventilation, the volume of air inhaled or exhaled per minute, rises significantly during pregnancy. This increase is primarily driven by an elevation in tidal volume (the amount of air inhaled or exhaled with each breath), rather than an increase in respiratory rate. The rise in minute ventilation supports the higher oxygen demand and helps remove carbon dioxide from the maternal bloodstream.

Hormonal Influence: Hormones, such as progesterone, estrogen, and relaxin, play a role in respiratory adaptations during pregnancy. These hormones relax the smooth muscles of the respiratory tract, resulting in improved airway diameter and reduced airway resistance.

Pregnancy induces remarkable adaptations in the cardiovascular and respiratory systems to support the metabolic needs of the mother and the developing foetus. These adaptations include increased blood volume, enhanced cardiac output, changes in heart rate and blood pressure, as well as increased oxygen demand, altered breathing pattern, elevated minute ventilation, and hormonal influences on the respiratory system. Understanding these physiological changes is crucial for healthcare providers to monitor and manage the health of pregnant women effectively.

Weight gain and distribution

During pregnancy, weight gain is a natural and necessary part of the process as the body prepares to support the growth and development of the baby. However, the amount of weight gained and how it is distributed can vary among individuals. Here are some key points regarding weight gain and distribution during pregnancy:

Recommended Weight Gain: The Institute of Medicine (IOM) provides guidelines for weight gain during pregnancy based on a woman's pre-pregnancy body mass index (BMI). The recommendations are as follows:

Underweight (BMI less than 18.5): 28-40 pounds (12.5-18 kg)
Normal weight (BMI 18.5-24.9): 25-35 pounds (11.5-16 kg)
Overweight (BMI 25-29.9): 15-25 pounds (7-11.5 kg)
Obese (BMI greater than or equal to 30): 11-20 pounds (5-9 kg)
You have to note that these are general guidelines, and individual variations exist. It is advisable to consult with a healthcare provider for your recommendations.

Distribution of Weight Gain: Weight gain during pregnancy is not just limited to the baby's weight. It includes several components:

Baby: The baby's weight is a significant contributor to overall weight gain. On average, a full-term baby weighs around 7-8 pounds (3.2-3.6 kg).

Placenta: The placenta, which provides nutrients and oxygen to the baby, typically weighs around 1.5 pounds (0.7 kg).

Amniotic Fluid: Amniotic fluid, which surrounds and cushions the baby, weighs approximately 2 pounds (0.9 kg).

Increased Blood Volume: During pregnancy, blood volume increases to support the needs of the developing baby. This can contribute to an increase in weight, amounting to about 4 pounds (1.8 kg).

Breast Tissue: The breasts undergo changes in preparation for breastfeeding, leading to an increase in their size and weight. This can account for around 2-3 pounds (0.9-1.4 kg).

Maternal Fat Stores: The body stores additional fat to provide energy reserves for pregnancy and breastfeeding. The amount of fat gained varies but can range from 4-8 pounds (1.8-3.6 kg).

Individual Variations: It's important to remember that every woman's body is unique, and weight gain during pregnancy can vary. Some women may gain more weight in certain areas, such as the abdomen, hips, and thighs, while others may distribute it more evenly throughout the body. Factors like genetics, body composition, and overall health can influence how weight is distributed.

Healthy Weight Management: Maintaining a healthy weight during pregnancy is crucial for the well-being of both the mother and the baby. It's advisable to follow a balanced and nutritious diet, engage in regular physical activity (with the guidance of a healthcare provider), and monitor weight gain as per the recommendations provided by the healthcare team.

Remember, weight gain during pregnancy is a natural and necessary part of the process. However, excessive weight gain or inadequate weight gain can pose risks to the health of both the mother and the baby. Regular prenatal care, including discussions with healthcare providers, can help ensure appropriate weight gain and address any concerns or questions throughout the pregnancy journey.

CHAPTER 2

NURTURING A HEALTHY MINDSET

Embracing body image changes

Pregnancy brings about numerous physical changes, both visible and internal. From weight gain and a growing belly to swollen ankles and hormonal fluctuations, your body is working hard to create a nurturing environment for your little one. While these changes may sometimes feel overwhelming or unfamiliar, it's essential to remember that they are natural and temporary.

One of the most crucial aspects of embracing body image changes during pregnancy is cultivating self-acceptance and self-love. Your body is performing an extraordinary feat, and every shift it undergoes is a testament to the miracle of life. Instead of focusing on societal ideals or comparing yourself to others, remind yourself that your body is doing exactly what it needs to do to support the growth and development of your baby.

Surround yourself with positive influences and supportive individuals who understand and appreciate the beauty of pregnancy. Seek out communities, whether online or in-person, where you can connect with other expectant mothers who are going through similar experiences. Sharing your thoughts, concerns, and joys with like-minded individuals can help normalize the changes you're experiencing and provide a valuable support system.

Practicing self-care is another crucial aspect of embracing body image changes during pregnancy. Treat yourself with kindness and compassion. Engage in activities that make you feel good, whether it's taking relaxing baths, practicing gentle prenatal yoga, or indulging in healthy and nourishing foods. Remember that self-care is not selfish; it's a vital part of maintaining your physical and emotional well-being throughout your pregnancy journey.

It's also worth noting that your body will gradually return to its pre-pregnancy state after you give birth. It may take time, and every individual's journey is unique, but it's important to be patient with yourself. Your body has undergone incredible changes, and it will require time to adjust and heal. Embracing your postpartum body with the same love and acceptance as you did during pregnancy is essential for your overall well-being.

Lastly, keep in mind that your body image does not define your worth as a mother or as a person. Your love, care, and nurturing are what truly matter. Focus on the joy and excitement of welcoming a new life into the world, and remember that your body's changes are a testament to the incredible journey of motherhood.

Embrace these body image changes with confidence, love, and gratitude. Celebrate the unique beauty that comes with pregnancy, and cherish this remarkable time in your life.

Managing pregnancy-related anxiety

Pregnancy is a time of significant physical and emotional changes, and it is not uncommon for expectant mothers to experience anxiety during this period. Pregnancy-related anxiety can arise from various factors, such as concerns about the health of the baby, fear of childbirth, changes in body image, financial worries, or the pressure of becoming a parent. It is essential to address and manage this anxiety to ensure the well-being of both the mother and the baby. Here are some strategies to help manage pregnancy-related anxiety:

Educate Yourself: Knowledge about pregnancy, childbirth, and the changes happening in your body can help alleviate anxiety. Attend prenatal classes, read books, and consult reliable sources to understand what to expect during each stage of pregnancy. This information can empower you and provide reassurance.

Communicate: Share your concerns and fears with your partner, family, or close friends. Talking about your anxieties can provide emotional support and perspective. Consider joining support groups or online forums where you can connect with other expectant mothers and share experiences.

Seek Prenatal Care: Regular prenatal check-ups with your healthcare provider are very important. These appointments allow you to monitor the progress of your pregnancy, address any concerns, and receive guidance. Establishing a trusting relationship with your healthcare provider can help alleviate anxiety.

Practice Relaxation Techniques: Engage in relaxation techniques such as deep breathing, meditation, prenatal yoga, or gentle exercise. These activities can help reduce stress, promote emotional well-being, and improve sleep quality.

Prioritize Self-Care: Take care of your physical and emotional well-being by prioritizing self-care. Get adequate rest, maintain a balanced diet, engage in gentle physical activities suitable for pregnancy, and pamper yourself with activities you enjoy. Consider activities like reading, listening to soothing music, taking baths, or practicing mindfulness.

Manage Information Intake: While it's important to stay informed, excessive exposure to negative or anxiety-inducing information can worsen pregnancy-related anxiety. Limit your intake of news, social media, or stories that trigger anxiety.

Engage in Supportive Relationships: Surround yourself with supportive and understanding individuals. Seek the company of loved ones who can provide emotional support and encouragement throughout your pregnancy journey.

Consider Therapy: If your anxiety becomes overwhelming or persists, consider seeking professional help. Therapists or counselors experienced in perinatal mental health can provide valuable guidance and support. They can help you develop coping strategies, challenge negative thoughts, and manage anxiety effectively.

Remember, pregnancy-related anxiety is a common experience, and you are not alone. By implementing these strategies and seeking support when needed, you can better manage anxiety and promote a healthy and positive pregnancy experience.

Building confidence in your changing abilities

It's natural to have concerns about the changes happening in your body and how they may affect your abilities. However, remember that you are strong and capable, and building confidence in your changing abilities is crucial for a positive pregnancy experience. Here are some tips to help you along this journey :

Educate Yourself: Knowledge is power. Take the time to learn about the different stages of pregnancy, the physical changes your body will undergo, and the various birthing options available to you. Understanding the natural processes taking place will help you feel more confident in your body's ability to adapt and nurture a growing life.

Stay Active: Regular physical activity during pregnancy can have numerous benefits. Engage in activities that are safe and suitable for your stage of pregnancy, such as prenatal yoga, swimming, or walking. Exercise not only helps maintain your physical health but also boosts your mental well-being and self-confidence.

Seek Support: Surround yourself with a supportive network of family, friends, and healthcare professionals who can offer guidance, encouragement, and reassurance. Joining prenatal classes or support groups allows you to connect with other expecting parents who may be going through similar experiences.

Practice Self-Care: Take care of your physical appearance and emotional well-being. Get enough rest, eat nutritious meals, and try to always stay hydrated. Engage in activities that help you relax and reduce stress, such as reading, meditating, taking baths, or listening to soothing music. When you prioritize self-care, you'll feel more confident in your ability to navigate the challenges that come with pregnancy.

Embrace Changes: Pregnancy brings about many physical changes, both visible and internal. Embrace these changes as signs of the incredible journey you're on. Celebrate the growing life within you and focus on the miraculous abilities of your body. Remember, every woman's pregnancy experience is unique, and your body is doing exactly what it needs to do to support your baby's growth.

Trust Yourself: You are the expert on your own body. Trust your instincts and listen to what your body is telling you. If something is wrong, don't hesitate to reach out to your healthcare provider for guidance. Trusting yourself and your intuition will help you make informed decisions and feel confident in your ability to care for yourself and your baby.

Practice Positive Affirmations: Surround yourself with positive thoughts and affirmations. Remind yourself daily of your strength, resilience, and ability to handle whatever comes your way. Repeat affirmations such as,

"I trust my body's wisdom," "I am capable of birthing my baby," or "I embrace the changes in my body with love and acceptance." These positive messages can help build your confidence and reinforce a healthy mindset.

Remember, building confidence in your changing abilities during pregnancy is an ongoing process. Be patient with yourself and allow yourself to experience the full range of emotions that come with this transformative time. Each day, remind yourself of your unique strengths, and believe in the incredible abilities that lie within you. You've got this!

connecting with your baby through exercise

One wonderful method to establish a deep bond and promote overall well-being is through exercise. Engaging in physical activities during pregnancy not only benefits your own health but also provides an opportunity for you to connect with your baby on a profound level.

Here are some ways in which exercise can help you connect with your baby during pregnancy:

Physical Sensations: When you exercise, you become more aware of your body and its movements. As you engage in activities like yoga, swimming, or gentle aerobics, you can consciously direct your attention towards your baby. Focus on the physical sensations you experience during exercise, such as the gentle kicks or movements your baby makes in response to your own motions. This heightened awareness can create a beautiful connection between you and your little one.

Mindful Movement: Exercise can be a meditative practice that allows you to be fully present in the moment. By incorporating mindfulness techniques into your workouts, you can cultivate a deep sense of connection with your baby. As you engage in activities like walking, dancing, or prenatal yoga, bring your attention to your baby, imagining their presence and sending them love and positive energy with each movement.

Bonding Hormones: Physical activity releases endorphins and various hormones that uplift your mood and create a sense of well-being. These hormones, such as oxytocin and serotonin, not only benefit your emotional state but also have the potential to influence your baby's environment. As you exercise, these hormones can traverse the placenta, positively affecting your baby's mood and development. This shared hormonal experience can foster a strong bond between you and your little one.

Shared Rhythm: Engaging in rhythmic activities like prenatal dance or gentle swaying can create a shared rhythm between you and your baby. Your movements can provide a soothing and comforting experience for your baby, as they feel the gentle sways and motions in the womb. This synchronized rhythm can foster a sense of connection and harmony between you both.

Relaxation and Stress Reduction: Pregnancy often brings about physical discomfort and emotional changes. Regular exercise helps to alleviate stress, reduce anxiety, and promote relaxation. When you are calm and relaxed, it creates a serene environment for your baby. Through exercise, you can create a tranquil space for both of you, enhancing your connection and promoting overall well-being.

Remember to consult with your healthcare provider before starting or continuing any exercise regimen during pregnancy. They can provide personalized recommendations based on your specific needs and any underlying medical conditions.

Take the time to connect with your baby through exercise during pregnancy. Embrace the journey, listen to your body, and cherish these precious moments as you build a strong bond that will last a lifetime.

CHAPTER 3:

SAFETY PRECAUTIONS AND GUIDELINES

Consulting with your healthcare provider

During pregnancy, it is crucial to maintain regular contact and consult with your healthcare provider to ensure a healthy pregnancy and the well-being of both you and your baby. Regular prenatal care is essential for monitoring the progress of your pregnancy, detecting any potential complications, and receiving appropriate guidance and support. Here are some key reasons why consulting with your healthcare provider is important during pregnancy:

Confirming Pregnancy: The first step is to schedule an appointment with your healthcare provider to confirm your pregnancy through a clinical assessment and, if necessary, a pregnancy test. This initial consultation helps establish a baseline for your prenatal care.

Monitoring Pregnancy Progress: Regular check-ups throughout your pregnancy allow your healthcare provider to monitor your baby's growth and development. They will measure your blood pressure, track weight gain, check the baby's heart rate, and perform other necessary tests to ensure a healthy progression.

Managing Health Conditions: If you have any pre-existing health conditions, such as diabetes, hypertension, or thyroid disorders, your healthcare provider will guide you on managing these conditions during pregnancy. They will help adjust medications, monitor your condition closely, and provide necessary guidance to ensure optimal health for both you and your baby.

Detecting and Preventing Complications: Routine prenatal visits enable your healthcare provider to identify any potential complications early on. Through various screenings and tests, such as blood tests, ultrasounds, and genetic screenings, they can detect conditions like gestational diabetes, preeclampsia, or birth defects. Early detection allows for timely interventions and appropriate management.

Nutrition and Lifestyle Guidance: Your healthcare provider will offer guidance on maintaining a healthy diet, including essential nutrients for you and your growing baby. They will also advise on safe exercise routines, adequate rest, and avoiding harmful substances like tobacco, alcohol, or certain medications that may pose risks during pregnancy.

Addressing Pregnancy Discomforts: Pregnancy often brings various discomforts such as morning sickness, back pain, or swollen ankles. Your healthcare provider can provide strategies to alleviate these discomforts, recommend safe over-the-counter medications, or suggest alternative therapies to promote your comfort.

Emotional Support and Education: Your healthcare provider plays a vital role in addressing your emotional well-being during pregnancy. They can offer reassurance, answer questions, and provide educational resources to help you navigate the physical and emotional changes you experience.

Birth Planning: Consulting with your healthcare provider allows you to discuss your birth preferences, understand available birthing options, and develop a birth plan tailored to your needs. They can also help you understand the signs of labor and when to seek medical assistance.

Remember, open and honest communication with your healthcare provider is essential. Share any concerns, ask questions, and actively participate in discussions regarding your pregnancy. Their expertise and guidance will help ensure a healthy and positive pregnancy experience for you and your baby.

Identifying warning signs and red flags

Pregnancy is a precious time in a woman's life, but it is essential to monitor one's health throughout this journey. While most pregnancies progress smoothly, it is crucial to be aware of warning signs and red flags that may indicate potential complications. Identifying and addressing these signs promptly can help ensure the well-being of both the mother and the baby. In this note, we will discuss some common warning signs and red flags that expectant mothers should be vigilant about during pregnancy.

Vaginal bleeding:
Any form of vaginal bleeding during pregnancy should be considered a warning sign. It can indicate several conditions, such as ectopic pregnancy, miscarriage, or placental problems. Even light spotting should not be ignored and should be reported to a healthcare professional.

Severe abdominal pain:
Experiencing intense abdominal pain could be a red flag. It might indicate conditions such as ectopic pregnancy, miscarriage, placental abruption, or preterm labor. Persistent or severe abdominal pain should be evaluated by a healthcare provider immediately.

Decreased fetal movement:

Feeling decreased fetal movement can be a potential red flag, especially during the third trimester. If a pregnant woman notices a significant decrease in fetal movements, she should seek medical attention to ensure the baby's well-being.

Severe or persistent headaches:
While headaches are common during pregnancy, severe or persistent headaches can indicate conditions like preeclampsia. High blood pressure, accompanied by other symptoms like visual disturbances and swelling, warrants immediate medical evaluation.

Swelling:
Swelling of the hands, face, legs, or ankles can be normal during pregnancy. However, sudden or excessive swelling, especially accompanied by other symptoms like high blood pressure, could be a sign of preeclampsia. It is crucial to report such swelling to a healthcare professional.

Vision changes:
Blurred vision, seeing spots or flashing lights, or any other significant changes in vision should not be ignored. These symptoms can be indicative of preeclampsia or other vision-related issues that require medical attention.

Persistent vomiting or nausea:
While morning sickness is common in the early stages of pregnancy, persistent vomiting or nausea that lasts

throughout the day and affects the woman's ability to eat or drink can be a sign of hyperemesis gravidarum. This condition may lead to dehydration and nutritional deficiencies and should be addressed by a healthcare provider.

Preterm labor signs:
Recognizing the signs of preterm labor is crucial for timely intervention. Warning signs include regular contractions before 37 weeks, lower back pain, pelvic pressure, abdominal cramping, or a sudden increase in vaginal discharge. If any of these symptoms occur, it is important to contact a healthcare professional immediately.
Pregnancy is a transformative journey, and being aware of warning signs and red flags is vital for ensuring a healthy pregnancy. This note has highlighted some common signs that expectant mothers should pay attention to and seek medical advice if they experience any of them. Regular prenatal care and open communication with healthcare providers are essential for monitoring and addressing potential complications, promoting the well-being of both the mother and the baby.

Modifying exercise routines for each trimester

Exercise during pregnancy can provide numerous benefits, such as improved cardiovascular health, increased strength and endurance, better mood, and enhanced overall well-being. However, as the body undergoes significant changes during each trimester, it's crucial to modify exercise routines accordingly to ensure the safety and comfort of both the mother and the developing baby. Here are some general guidelines for modifying exercise routines during each trimester of pregnancy:

First Trimester (Weeks 1-12):

Consult with your healthcare provider: Before starting or continuing an exercise program, it is important to consult with your healthcare provider to ensure you have medical clearance and discuss any specific considerations based on your health and pregnancy.

Listen to your body: Pay attention to how your body reacts during exercise. If you experience any unusual symptoms such as dizziness, shortness of breath, pain, or excessive fatigue, stop exercising and consult with your healthcare provider.

Focus on low-impact activities: Engage in exercises that are low-impact and gentle on your joints, such as walking, swimming, stationary cycling, prenatal yoga, or prenatal Pilates. These activities help maintain cardiovascular fitness and muscular strength without placing excessive stress on your body.

Avoid exercises that involve lying flat on your back: As your pregnancy progresses, lying flat on your back can compress a major vein called the vena cava, reducing blood flow to the uterus and potentially causing dizziness. Opt for exercises performed in a side-lying position or with an incline.

Second Trimester (Weeks 13-27):

Continue with low-impact exercises: Continue engaging in low-impact exercises like walking, swimming, and prenatal yoga. These activities help promote circulation, maintain muscle tone, and support good posture.

Modify abdominal exercises: Avoid traditional crunches or exercises that put excessive strain on the abdominal muscles. Instead, focus on exercises that strengthen the core and pelvic floor, such as Kegels and modified planks. Consider seeking guidance from a certified prenatal fitness instructor.

Use proper body mechanics: Pay attention to your body mechanics during exercise to protect your joints and maintain stability. Avoid sudden jerky movements, and be mindful of balance and coordination as your center of gravity shifts.

Wear supportive clothing and footwear: Invest in comfortable, supportive maternity workout clothes and properly fitted athletic shoes to provide adequate support to your changing body and help prevent discomfort or injury.

Third Trimester (Weeks 28-40+):

Prioritize safety and comfort: As you approach the end of your pregnancy, focus on exercises that are safe and comfortable. Low-impact activities such as walking, swimming, and prenatal yoga can continue to be beneficial.

Modify intensity and duration: Reduce the intensity and duration of your workouts, as your body requires more energy to support the growing baby. Shorter, frequent exercise sessions may be more manageable than longer ones.

Use props and support: Incorporate props like pillows or exercise balls to support your body and help maintain proper alignment during exercises. These props can also provide added stability and comfort during stretching or relaxation exercises.

Stay hydrated and avoid overheating: Pregnancy increases the body's need for hydration. Drink plenty of water before, during, and after exercise, and avoid exercising in hot or humid environments to prevent overheating.

Remember, every pregnancy is unique, and it is essential to consult with your healthcare provider and follow their guidance when modifying your exercise routine. They can provide personalized advice based on your health, fitness level, and any specific considerations related to your pregnancy.

Staying hydrated and maintaining proper nutrition

Staying hydrated and maintaining proper nutrition are essential aspects of a healthy pregnancy. Here are some important points to note down:

Hydration:

Drink plenty of water: Aim for at least 8-10 cups (64-80 ounces) of water per day. Proper hydration helps maintain amniotic fluid levels and supports healthy blood circulation.

Avoid sugary drinks: Opt for water, herbal teas, or natural fruit-infused water instead of sugary beverages, as excessive sugar intake can lead to unnecessary weight gain and potential complications.

Monitor urine color: Your urine should be light yellow or clear. Dark yellow urine may indicate dehydration, so drink more fluids if this occurs.

Stay cool: Pregnant women are more prone to overheating. Carry a water bottle with you and avoid excessive heat exposure.

Nutritional Guidelines:

Eat a balanced diet: Focus on whole foods such as fruits, vegetables, whole grains, lean proteins, and healthy fats. Include a variety of colors on your plate to ensure a wide range of nutrients.

Folic acid and iron: These are vital for fetal development and preventing birth defects. Incorporate foods like leafy greens, beans, fortified cereals, and lean meats into your diet.

Calcium-rich foods: Ensure adequate intake of dairy products, tofu, almonds, and leafy greens for healthy bone development in your baby.

Omega-3 fatty acids: These are essential for the baby's brain and eye development. Include fatty fish (like salmon), chia seeds, walnuts, and flaxseeds in your meals.

Avoid excess caffeine and processed foods: Limit your intake of caffeine, as high amounts may increase the risk of miscarriage. Minimize processed foods, sugary snacks, and empty calories to maintain optimal nutrition.

Small, frequent meals:

Opt for 5-6 smaller meals throughout the day instead of three large meals. This helps prevent indigestion, nausea, and bloating, which are common during pregnancy.

Snack wisely: Choose nutrient-dense snacks like yogurt, fresh fruits, nuts, and whole-grain crackers to keep your energy levels up and provide essential nutrients between meals.

Consult your healthcare provider:

Every pregnancy is unique, and nutritional requirements might be different. Regularly consult your healthcare provider for personalized advice and to address any specific concerns or dietary restrictions you may have. Remember, maintaining proper hydration and nutrition during pregnancy is vital for your well-being and the healthy development of your baby. Embrace this special time and take care of yourself .

CHAPTER 4:

THE ESSENTIAL EXERCISES FOR PREGNANCY

Strengthening the pelvic floor

One crucial aspect of pregnancy that often goes unnoticed is the strengthening of the pelvic floor muscles. The pelvic floor plays a vital role in supporting the pelvic organs, maintaining bowel and bladder control, and facilitating a healthy delivery. Strengthening these muscles during pregnancy can contribute to your overall comfort, prevent complications, and aid in postpartum recovery.

Here are some key tips for strengthening the pelvic floor during pregnancy:

Kegel exercises: Kegels are the most commonly recommended exercises for strengthening the pelvic floor. They involve contracting and releasing the muscles that control urine flow.

Basic Kegels: Sit or lie down comfortably and squeeze the muscles around your vagina, as if you are trying to stop the flow of urine. Hold the contraction for some seconds, then release. Repeat this cycle 10-15 times, three times a day.

Elevator Kegels: Imagine your pelvic floor muscles as an elevator with different levels. Slowly contract and lift the muscles, as if you're moving the elevator up one level at a time. Pause briefly at each level before gradually releasing and lowering the muscles. Repeat this cycle 10-15 times.

Quick Kegels: Contract and release your pelvic floor muscles quickly, as if you are doing a rapid series of pulses. Do this for 10 seconds, then rest for 10 seconds. Repeat 10 times.

Bridge Kegels: Lie on your back with your knees bent and feet flat on the floor. Lift your hips from the ground, engaging your glutes and pelvic floor muscles. Hold for some few seconds, then slowly lower back down. Repeat this exercise 10-15 times.

Side-lying Kegels: Lie on your side with your knees slightly bent. Contract your pelvic floor muscles as you would for a regular Kegel exercise. Hold for a few seconds, then release. Repeat 10-15 times on each side.

Remember to breathe normally and avoid tensing other muscles while performing these exercises.

Pelvic tilts: Pelvic tilts help improve the flexibility and strength of the lower back and pelvic muscles. Start by standing with your back against a wall, feet shoulder-width apart. Slowly tilt your pelvis forward, pressing the small of your back against the wall. Hold for some seconds, then tilt your pelvis backwards. Repeat this exercise several times, focusing on controlled movements.

Squats: Squats are an excellent way to engage the pelvic floor muscles and strengthen the lower body. Stand with your feet shoulder-width apart and slowly lower your body into a squatting position. Keep your back straight and then your knees aligned with your toes. Hold the squat briefly, then rise back up. Start with a few repetitions and gradually increase as you feel comfortable.

Yoga and Pilates: Prenatal yoga and Pilates classes often include exercises that target the pelvic floor. These practices focus on gentle stretches, controlled movements, and breathing techniques that help strengthen and relax the pelvic floor muscles.
Yoga exercises during pregnancy:

Cat-Cow Stretch: Get on your hands and knees, with your hands aligned under your shoulders and knees under your hips. Inhale and lift your head and tallbone while dropping your belly towards the floor (Cow pose). Exhale and round your back,then tuck your chin towards your chest (Cat pose). Repeat this gentle flowing movement for a few rounds.

Modified Triangle Pose: Stand with your feet wide apart. Turn your right foot out and extend your arms out to your sides. Inhale and reach your right arm forward, then exhale and hinge at the hip, lowering your right hand to your shin or a block. Extend your left arm straight up towards the sky . Hold for some breaths and repeat on the other side.

Prenatal Sun Salutation: Start standing and bring your palms together at your heart center. Inhale, raise your arms overhead, and gently arch your back. Exhale, fold forward, bending your knees if needed. Inhale, lift halfway up, and place your hands on your shins. Exhale, step or gently hop back into a modified plank pose. Continue flowing through modified chaturanga, upward-facing dog, and downward-facing dog. Modify the movements as needed and listen to your body.

Pilates exercises during pregnancy:

Pelvic Tilts: Lie down on your back with your knees bent and your feet flat on the ground. Inhale, and as you exhale, tilt your pelvis upward, engaging your abdominal muscles and pressing your lower back into the floor. Inhale, release the tilt, and return to neutral. Repeat for a few rounds, focusing on controlled movements.

Arm and Leg Extensions: Start on your hands and knees, with your hands aligned under your shoulders and knees under your hips. Extend your right arm forward and your left leg backward, keeping them parallel to the floor. Hold for a few breaths, engaging your core for stability. Return to where you started from and do the same on the other side.

Modified Side Plank: Lie on your side with your bottom elbow directly beneath your shoulder, and your legs stacked on top of each other. Lift your hips off the floor, creating a straight line from your head to your feet. Modify by bending your bottom knee and placing your foot on the floor for added stability. Hold for a few breaths and change sides.

Consult with a physical therapist: If you're experiencing any pelvic floor issues or want personalized guidance, consider consulting with a physical therapist specializing in women's health. They can assess your specific needs and provide a tailored exercise program to strengthen your pelvic floor muscles safely and effectively.

Remember, it's crucial to listen to your body during pregnancy. If any exercise feels uncomfortable or causes pain, stop and consult your healthcare provider. Additionally, maintaining good posture, avoiding heavy lifting, and practicing proper body mechanics can also contribute to pelvic floor health.

Taking care of your pelvic floor during pregnancy is an investment in your long-term well-being. By incorporating these exercises into your daily routine, you can strengthen the pelvic floor muscles, reduce the risk of complications, and promote a smoother pregnancy and postpartum recovery.

Engaging the core muscles

Pregnancy is a transformative and exciting time for women. It's important to maintain overall fitness and well-being during this period, and engaging the core muscles can play a crucial role in supporting the body and minimizing discomfort. Core muscles include the muscles in the abdomen, back, and pelvis, and strengthening them can provide numerous benefits during pregnancy and postpartum. In this note, we will explore the significance of engaging core muscles during pregnancy and provide some safe exercises and tips to achieve a healthy core.

Benefits of Engaging Core Muscles:

Improved Stability: As the baby grows, the added weight can lead to an altered center of gravity, placing strain on the back and pelvis. Engaging the core muscles helps to stabilize the spine and pelvis, reducing the risk of pain and injury.

Reduced Back Pain: Pregnancy-related back pain is common due to the postural changes and increased stress on the spine. Strengthening the core can provide better support for the back and alleviate discomfort.

Enhanced Posture: As the abdominal muscles stretch to accommodate the growing baby, posture can be affected. Engaging the core muscles helps maintain proper alignment and reduces the tendency to slouch, promoting better posture and minimizing strain on the back.

Easier Labor and Delivery: Engaging the core muscles can improve overall strength, stamina, and endurance, which may contribute to a smoother labor and delivery experience.

Safe Exercises for Engaging Core Muscles:

Pelvic Floor Exercises: Kegels are a beneficial exercise for strengthening the pelvic floor muscles, which provide support to the uterus, bladder, and bowel. To perform Kegels, contract the muscles used to stop the flow of urine, hold for a few seconds, and then release. Repeat this exercise different times during the day.

Abdominal Bracing: This exercise involves gently contracting the deep abdominal muscles without holding the breath. Stand or sit with proper posture, imagine pulling the navel towards the spine, and hold for a few seconds before releasing. Repeat this exercise throughout the day.

Modified Plank: Start on all fours, aligning the wrists under the shoulders and the knees under the hips. Extend one leg back, keeping it straight, and then extend the opposite arm forward. Let the neutral spine be maintained and engage the core muscles. Hold for a few seconds and then switch sides. Perform this exercise with caution and stop if it causes any discomfort.

Tips for Engaging Core Muscles Safely:

Consult a healthcare professional: Before starting any exercise program during pregnancy, it is essential to consult with a healthcare provider to ensure it is safe for your specific situation.

Listen to your body: Pay attention to your body's cues and modify or stop any exercise that causes pain, discomfort, or excessive fatigue.

Avoid lying flat on your back: As pregnancy progresses, lying flat on your back for extended periods can compress major blood vessels and reduce blood flow to the uterus. Opt for exercises performed in an elevated or inclined position.

Practice diaphragmatic breathing: Breathing deeply using the diaphragm helps activate the core muscles while providing relaxation and oxygenation. Inhale deeply, allowing the abdomen to expand, and exhale fully, drawing the navel gently towards the spine.

Engaging the core muscles during pregnancy offers a range of benefits, including improved stability, reduced back pain, enhanced posture, and potential benefits during labor and delivery. Remember to always consult with a healthcare provider before starting or modifying any exercise routine during pregnancy. By incorporating safe exercises and techniques into your fitness regimen, you can support your body's changes, maintain optimal well-being, and prepare for the journey of motherhood.

Working the upper body

Maintaining a regular exercise routine during pregnancy can be beneficial for your overall well-being, including your upper body strength. However, it's crucial to prioritize safety and listen to your body's needs throughout each trimester. Here are some important points to note down :

Consult with your healthcare provider: Before beginning or continuing any exercise program during pregnancy, it's important to consult with your healthcare provider. They can provide personalized advice based on your medical history and the specific needs of your pregnancy.

Focus on low-impact exercises: As your body undergoes changes to accommodate your growing baby, it's generally recommended to focus on low-impact exercises that minimize stress on your joints. Examples of suitable upper body exercises include seated or supported arm exercises, resistance band workouts, and gentle stretching routines.

Be mindful of posture and alignment: Pregnancy can affect your posture due to the shifting center of gravity and increased weight in the front of your body. Pay attention to your posture during upper body exercises to maintain proper alignment and reduce strain on your back and shoulders. Avoid exercises that involve heavy weights or put excessive pressure on your abdominal area.

Modify exercises as needed: As your pregnancy progresses, you may need to modify certain exercises to accommodate the changes in your body. For example, you might consider using lighter weights or opting for bodyweight exercises instead. Additionally, avoid exercises that require lying flat on your back after the first trimester, as this position can restrict blood flow to the baby.

Don't overexert yourself: Pregnancy is not the time to push your limits or strive for new personal records. Instead, focus on maintaining your current fitness level and staying active within a comfortable range. Overexertion can lead to fatigue, dizziness, and potentially harm you or your baby.

Stay hydrated and take breaks: It's crucial to stay hydrated during exercise, especially when pregnant. Be sure to drink plenty of water before, during, and after your workouts. Additionally, listen to your body and take breaks as it is needed. If you feel fatigued or short of breath, take a rest and resume exercise when you're ready.

Remember, every pregnancy is unique, and it's essential to honor your body's needs and limitations. If you experience any discomfort, pain, or unusual symptoms during or after exercising, stop and consult your healthcare provider immediately.

Lower body strength and stability

During pregnancy, maintaining lower body strength and stability is crucial for the overall well-being and comfort of expectant mothers. Strong and stable lower body muscles provide support, help alleviate common pregnancy discomforts, and facilitate safe movements throughout the various stages of pregnancy. Here are some important points to consider at this point :

Importance of Lower Body Strength: Pregnancy places additional stress on a woman's body, particularly in the lower back, hips, and pelvis. Strengthening the lower body muscles, including the glutes, quadriceps, hamstrings, and calves, can help alleviate discomfort and improve posture and stability.

Benefits of Lower Body Strength and Stability:

Reduced back pain: Strengthening the muscles in the lower back and hips can alleviate the strain caused by the growing belly and shifting center of gravity.
Improved balance: As the pregnancy progresses, changes in weight distribution can affect balance. Strengthening the lower body muscles helps maintain stability and reduces the risk of falls.
Easier labor and delivery: Strengthening the pelvic floor and lower body muscles can enhance endurance, support the baby's descent, and aid in pushing during labor.

Postpartum recovery: Maintaining lower body strength during pregnancy can contribute to a faster recovery after childbirth.

Safe Exercises for Lower Body Strength and Stability:

Squats: Stand with your feet shoulder-width apart and slowly lower yourself into a squatting position, keeping your back straight and your knees in line with your toes. Hold that position for some few seconds and then slowly rise back up. This exercise helps strengthen the glutes, thighs, and pelvic floor muscles.

Lunges: Take a step forward with one leg, bending both knees to a 90-degree angle. Push back up to the position you started from and repeat on the other leg. Lunges work the quadriceps, hamstrings, and glutes while also improving balance and stability.

Wall sits: Stand with your back against a wall and then slowly slide down until your knees are bent at a 90-degree angle. Hold this position for as long as you can comfortably manage, and then slowly push back up. Wall sits help strengthen the thighs and glutes.

Pelvic tilts: Stand with your back against a wall and then your feet shoulder-width apart. Slowly tilt your pelvis forward and backward, focusing on engaging your abdominal muscles and maintaining a neutral spine. This exercise helps strengthen the core and stabilize the lower back.

Step-ups: Find a sturdy step or platform and step up onto it with one foot, then bring the other foot up to join it. Step back down and repeat with the other foot in front. Step-ups engage the glutes, quadriceps, and calves, and also help improve balance.

Glute bridges: Lie on your back with your knees bent and your feet flat on the ground. Engage your glutes and lift your hips off the ground, making them form a straight line from your knees to your shoulders. Hold for a few seconds, then slowly lower back to the ground. Glute bridges target the glutes, hamstrings, and lower back muscles.

Kegel exercises: Focusing on the pelvic floor muscles, Kegels enhance strength and stability, aiding in childbirth and postpartum recovery.
Safety Precautions:

- Consult with a healthcare provider before starting any exercise routine during pregnancy, especially if you have any complications or medical conditions.
- Avoid exercises that involve lying flat on your back after the first trimester, as this can restrict blood flow to the uterus.
- Use proper form and techniques during exercise to reduce the risk of injury.

- Stay hydrated and avoid overheating during workouts.

Remember, every pregnancy is unique, and what works for one woman may not be suitable for another. It's essential to listen to your body and modify or discontinue exercises if they cause any discomfort or pain. Working with a certified prenatal fitness professional can provide personalized guidance and ensure safe and effective exercises tailored to your needs.

Stay active, prioritize your safety and well-being, and enjoy the benefits of maintaining lower body strength and stability throughout your pregnancy journey.

Enhancing flexibility and balance

Maintaining flexibility and balance during pregnancy can contribute to a more comfortable and healthy experience. Here are some tips to help you enhance flexibility and balance during this special time:

Consult your healthcare provider: Before engaging in any exercise routine, consult with your healthcare provider to ensure it is safe for you and your baby. He or she can provide personalized advice based on your individual needs and medical history.

Gentle stretching exercises: Incorporate gentle stretching exercises into your daily routine. Focus on areas prone to tightness, such as the neck, shoulders, lower back, hips, and legs. Stretching can help alleviate muscle tension and improve flexibility.

Prenatal yoga: Consider joining a prenatal yoga class or following online tutorials designed specifically for pregnant women. Prenatal yoga can help improve flexibility, balance, and posture while providing relaxation techniques and breath control.

Pelvic floor exercises: Strengthening your pelvic floor muscles is crucial during pregnancy and can assist with balance and stability. Perform Kegel exercises regularly to enhance the strength of these muscles. Consult a healthcare professional or a specialized prenatal exercise instructor for guidance.

Aqua aerobics: Water exercises, such as aqua aerobics, are excellent for improving flexibility and balance while minimizing strain on your joints. The buoyancy of water provides gentle resistance, making it a safe and effective option for pregnant women.

Mind-body practices: Explore mind-body practices such as tai chi or meditation. These practices can help improve balance, posture, and mental well-being during pregnancy. Engaging in mindful movements can enhance your body awareness and stability.

Supportive footwear: Wear comfortable and supportive footwear that provides stability and balance. As your pregnancy progresses, your center of gravity shifts, and wearing proper shoes can help prevent falls and support your posture.

Maintain good posture: Be careful of your posture throughout the day. Stand tall, keep your shoulders relaxed, and avoid slouching. Good posture can help maintain balance and prevent unnecessary strain on your body.

Use support aids: Consider using support aids, such as a pregnancy support belt or cushions, to provide additional support to your growing belly and alleviate strain on your back and hips.

Listen to your body: Always take heed to your body and respect its limits. Pregnancy is a unique journey for each woman, and what works for one may not work for another. If you feel any discomfort or pain during exercises, modify or stop the activity and consult your healthcare provider.

Remember, the goal is to maintain a healthy level of flexibility and balance throughout your pregnancy. By incorporating these tips into your daily routine, you can enhance your physical well-being, reduce discomfort, and prepare your body for childbirth. Enjoy this incredible time and take care of yourself and your growing baby.

chapter 5:

CARDIOVASCULAR FITNESS FOR EXPECTANT MOTHERS

Low-impact cardiovascular activities

During pregnancy, engaging in regular physical activity is beneficial for both the mother and the developing baby. Low-impact cardiovascular activities can provide numerous health advantages without placing excessive stress on the body. These activities help maintain cardiovascular fitness, improve overall well-being, and may aid in managing some pregnancy-related discomforts. However, it is crucial to consult with a healthcare professional before starting or continuing any exercise regimen during pregnancy.

Walking: Walking is a safe and effective low-impact activity that can be easily incorporated into daily routines. It helps improve cardiovascular health, strengthens leg muscles, and boosts mood. It's good you start with short walks and gradually increase the duration and intensity as tolerated.

Swimming: Swimming and water aerobics are excellent choices that can help during pregnancy. The buoyancy of water reduces the impact on joints and offers a full-body workout. These activities help alleviate swelling, reduce back pain, and promote cardiovascular fitness without straining the body.

Prenatal yoga: Prenatal yoga focuses on gentle stretching, relaxation, and breathing exercises. It helps improve flexibility, balance, and posture. Prenatal yoga classes are specifically designed to cater to the needs of pregnant women and often include modifications for various stages of pregnancy.

Stationary cycling: Using a stationary bike or participating in a spinning class provides a low-impact cardiovascular workout. It helps strengthen leg muscles, maintain cardiovascular fitness, and minimizes stress on the joints. Adjust the resistance and speed according to comfort level and avoid excessive strain.

Low-impact aerobics: Participating in low-impact aerobic classes or following suitable exercise videos designed for pregnant women can be beneficial. These workouts typically involve rhythmic movements that improve heart health, circulation, and stamina. Avoid high-impact moves, jumps, or sudden directional changes.

Prenatal dance classes: Prenatal dance classes, such as Zumba or other dance-based fitness programs designed for pregnant women, offer a fun and engaging way to stay active. They help enhance cardiovascular fitness, coordination, and flexibility. Ensure the movements are low-impact and avoid excessive twisting or jumping.

Remember these general guidelines when engaging in low-impact cardiovascular activities during pregnancy:

- Stay well-hydrated before, during, and after exercising.
- Wear comfortable clothing and supportive footwear.
- Warm up adequately with gentle stretching or light movements.
- Listen to your body and adjust the intensity or duration of the activity as needed.
- Avoid overheating and exercise in a well-ventilated environment.
- Incorporate proper posture and body mechanics to prevent strain or injury.
- Stop exercising if experiencing dizziness, shortness of breath, chest pain, vaginal bleeding, or any other concerning symptoms. Consult a healthcare professional immediately.

Every pregnancy is unique, and it's crucial to consult with a healthcare provider before starting or continuing any exercise routine. They can provide personalized recommendations based on your specific circumstances and medical history.

Safe and effective walking and jogging

During pregnancy, staying active through regular exercise is beneficial for both the mother and the baby. Walking and jogging are two low-impact activities that can be safe and effective options for expectant mothers. However, it's important to take certain precautions and listen to your body to ensure a safe and enjoyable exercise routine. Here are some guidelines for safe and effective walking and jogging during pregnancy:

Consult with your healthcare provider: Before starting any exercise routine, it's crucial to consult your healthcare provider. They can evaluate your individual situation and provide personalized advice based on your health, any complications, or specific needs during pregnancy.

Start gradually: If you're new to walking or jogging, begin with a comfortable pace and gradually increase your intensity and duration over time. It's recommended to aim for at least 150 minutes of moderate-intensity aerobic exercise spread throughout the week.

Wear appropriate footwear: Invest in a good pair of supportive and comfortable athletic shoes that provide adequate cushioning and stability. Pregnancy can affect the feet and ankles, so having proper footwear can reduce discomfort and minimize the risk of injury.

Warm-up and cool-down: Prior to each session, warm up your body with gentle stretches or light walking to prepare your muscles for exercise. Similarly, end your workout with a cool-down period to gradually lower your heart rate and help prevent muscle soreness.

Maintain good posture: Pay attention to your posture while walking or jogging. Keep your head up and shoulders relaxed, and then back straight. Avoid slouching or leaning forward excessively, as it can strain your back and put additional pressure on your abdomen.

Stay hydrated: Pregnancy increases the body's need for fluids. Drink plenty of water before, during, and after your exercising to stay hydrated. Dehydration can cause dizziness, fatigue, and other complications.

Listen to your body: Pregnancy is a time when your body undergoes significant changes, so it's essential to pay attention to its signals. If you experience any pain, dizziness, shortness of breath, or vaginal bleeding, stop exercising and consult your healthcare provider immediately.

Choose safe environments: Opt for well-lit, smooth, and even surfaces for walking and jogging. Avoid routes with uneven terrain, potholes, or high traffic areas to minimize the risk of falls or accidents.

Modify as your pregnancy progresses: As your pregnancy advances, you may need to modify your exercise routine. The growing belly can affect your balance and shift your center of gravity. Consider reducing the intensity, shortening your workout duration, or switching to alternative low-impact exercises if needed.

Stay cool and comfortable: Pregnancy can make you more susceptible to overheating. Exercise in a cool, well-ventilated environment, and dress in breathable, loose-fitting clothing to allow proper air circulation. Avoid exercising in extreme weather conditions.

Remember, every pregnancy is unique, and what works for one pregnant woman may not work for the other. Be mindful of your body's limitations and adjust your exercise routine accordingly. Regular walking and jogging, when done safely and effectively, can contribute to your overall well-being and promote a healthy pregnancy.

Swimming and aquatic exercises

Swimming and aquatic exercises can be highly beneficial for expectant mothers throughout their pregnancy. Engaging in these activities not only provides physical fitness but also promotes overall well-being. Here are some key points to write down:

Low-impact exercise: Swimming is a low-impact activity that puts minimal stress on joints and ligaments. This makes it an ideal form of exercise for expectant mothers who may experience discomfort or joint pain due to the additional weight of pregnancy.

Cardiovascular fitness: Swimming is a very good way that helps to improve cardiovascular fitness. It increases heart rate and lung capacity, enhancing circulation and oxygen flow to both the mother and the baby. Improved cardiovascular health can help alleviate pregnancy-related symptoms such as swelling and fatigue.

Muscle strengthening: Swimming engages various muscle groups, providing a full-body workout. It strengthens the arms, legs, back, and core muscles. This can help expectant mothers maintain muscle tone, improve posture, and alleviate back pain, which is common during pregnancy.

Weight control and fluid retention: Swimming can help manage weight gain during pregnancy by burning calories. It also aids in reducing fluid retention and swelling, as the water pressure helps to alleviate pressure on the joints and can assist with blood circulation.

Improved mood and reduced stress: Engaging in aquatic exercises has a positive impact on mental well-being. The buoyancy and calming effect of water can help alleviate stress, anxiety, and mood swings that are often experienced during pregnancy.

Reduced risk of overheating: Water helps regulate body temperature, reducing the risk of overheating during exercise. This is particularly important for pregnant women, as they are more prone to heat-related discomfort.

Safety precautions:
While swimming and aquatic exercises are generally safe for expectant mothers, it is essential to consult with a healthcare provider before starting any new exercise regimen. They can provide personalized advice based on individual health conditions and the stage of pregnancy.

Pool hygiene: It's important to choose swimming pools with proper hygiene and maintenance to minimize the risk of infections. Ensure that the pool water is adequately chlorinated and clean.

Water safety: When participating in aquatic exercises, it is crucial to prioritize safety. Always swim in designated areas, be mindful of depth, and avoid situations where there is a risk of slipping or falling.

In conclusion, swimming and aquatic exercises offer numerous benefits for expectant mothers. They provide a safe and effective way to stay active, strengthen muscles, improve cardiovascular health, and enhance overall well-being. However, it is essential to consult with a healthcare provider and follow safety guidelines to ensure a healthy and enjoyable experience.

Stationary cycling and elliptical training

Exercise during pregnancy is generally considered safe and beneficial for both the mother and the developing baby. Two popular forms of low-impact cardiovascular exercises often recommended during pregnancy are stationary cycling and elliptical training. However, it's essential to consult with your healthcare provider before starting any exercise program, as individual circumstances may vary.

Stationary Cycling:
Stationary cycling, also known as indoor cycling or spin classes, involves pedaling on a stationary bike. Here are some key points to note down :

a. Low impact: Stationary cycling is a low-impact exercise that puts minimal stress on the joints, making it suitable for pregnant women, especially those with joint discomfort or previous injuries.

b. Cardiovascular benefits: Cycling can improve cardiovascular health and endurance without excessive strain on the body. It helps strengthen the heart and lungs, promoting overall fitness during pregnancy.

c. Adjustable intensity: The intensity of stationary cycling can be easily adjusted according to your fitness level and comfort. You can control resistance, speed, and duration to tailor the workout to your needs.

d. Proper posture: Maintain an upright posture and avoid leaning too far forward to prevent strain on the back and pelvis. Adjust the bike's seat and handlebars to ensure proper alignment and support.

e. Safety precautions: Ensure the bike is stable and secure before each session. Stay hydrated, wear comfortable clothing, and use appropriate footwear. Listen to your body and stop if you experience any pain, dizziness, or shortness of breath.

Elliptical Training:
Elliptical training involves using a stationary machine that simulates walking or running while minimizing impact. Consider the following points when incorporating elliptical training into your pregnancy exercise routine:
a. Low impact: Similar to stationary cycling, elliptical training is gentle on the joints, reducing the risk of strain or injury during pregnancy.

b. Full-body workout: Elliptical machines engage both the upper and the lower body thus providing a well-rounded cardiovascular workout. It helps improve muscle tone and endurance while increasing heart rate without putting excessive stress on the body.

c. Balance and stability: As pregnancy progresses, the center of gravity shifts, affecting balance and stability. Using the elliptical machine's handles can provide additional support and stability, promoting safety during exercise.

d. Adjustable intensity: Elliptical machines usually offer adjustable resistance levels and incline settings. Start with a low intensity and gradually increase it as you feel comfortable. Pay attention to your body and avoid overexertion.

e. Safety precautions: Ensure the machine is in good working condition and properly maintained. Use supportive footwear, maintain good posture, and stay hydrated. Stop exercising if you experience any pain, discomfort, or signs of overexertion.

Remember that every pregnancy is unique, and individual circumstances may be different. Seek advice from your healthcare provider before starting or continuing any exercise program during pregnancy. They can provide personalized guidance based on your medical history and current health status.

It's important to listen to your body, take breaks when needed, and make modifications as your pregnancy progresses. Regular exercise can help promote overall well-being, maintain a healthy weight, alleviate pregnancy discomfort, and prepare you for childbirth.

Prenatal aerobic classes and dance workouts

Prenatal aerobic classes and dance workouts are popular and beneficial forms of exercise for pregnant women. These fitness activities not only help expectant mothers maintain a healthy lifestyle but also provide numerous physical and emotional advantages during pregnancy. Here are some important points to note down :

Physical Benefits:

Improved cardiovascular health: Aerobic exercises and dance workouts increase heart rate and circulation, enhancing overall cardiovascular fitness.
Increased endurance: Regular participation in prenatal aerobic classes and dance workouts can improve stamina and energy levels, which are particularly important during labor and delivery.
Strengthened muscles: These activities target major muscle groups, including the core, legs, and arms, helping to build strength and flexibility.
Enhanced balance and coordination: The movements and routines involved in dance workouts contribute to better balance and coordination, which can be especially beneficial as the body undergoes changes during pregnancy.
Weight management: Prenatal aerobic classes and dance workouts can assist in managing healthy weight gain during pregnancy and help prevent excessive weight gain.

Emotional Well-being:

Stress relief: Engaging in aerobic exercises and dance can serve as a form of stress relief, allowing pregnant women to release tension and boost their mood.
Increased energy and self-confidence: Regular physical activity promotes the release of endorphins, which are known to elevate mood and increase energy levels. This can contribute to improved self-confidence and a positive outlook.
Social support: Participating in prenatal aerobic classes and dance workouts often provides an opportunity to connect with other expectant mothers, creating a sense of community and support.

Safety Considerations:

Consultation with healthcare provider: Prior to starting any exercise program during pregnancy, it is crucial to consult with a healthcare provider. They can provide personalized advice based on individual health factors and ensure the chosen activities are suitable.
Modifications for pregnancy: Prenatal aerobic classes and dance workouts should be specifically designed or modified for pregnant women, taking into account the physiological changes and limitations that come with pregnancy.
Hydration and temperature regulation: Pregnant women should stay well-hydrated and avoid overheating during exercise. It is recommended to drink plenty of

water before, during, and after workouts and to exercise in a well-ventilated environment.

 Prenatal aerobic classes and dance workouts offer pregnant women a range of physical and emotional benefits. By promoting overall fitness, these activities can contribute to a healthier pregnancy, improved well-being, and potentially easier labor and delivery. However, it is essential to prioritize safety and consult with a healthcare provider to ensure that the chosen exercises are suitable for individual circumstances.

chapter 6

Adapting your fitness routine for each trimester

first trimester: navigating nausea and fatigue

As you enter the first trimester, it's important to adjust your fitness routine to accommodate the changes in your body. During this time, many women experience symptoms such as nausea and fatigue, which can make it challenging to maintain your regular exercise regimen. However, with a few modifications and mindful choices, you can continue to stay active and promote your overall well-being. Here are some tips for adapting your fitness routine during the first trimester while navigating nausea and fatigue:

Listen to your body: It's crucial to pay close attention to your body's signals and adjust your routine accordingly. If you're feeling excessively tired or nauseous, it's okay to take a break or reduce the intensity of your workouts. Rest is essential for your well-being and the development of your baby.

Choose gentle exercises: Opt for low-impact exercises that are gentle on your body, such as walking, swimming, or prenatal yoga. These activities can help improve circulation, maintain muscle tone, and promote relaxation without placing excessive stress on your joints.

Incorporate frequent breaks: Break up your exercise sessions into shorter intervals with frequent breaks to manage fatigue. This approach can help you maintain your energy levels and prevent overexertion. Aim for 10-15 minute sessions throughout the day rather than one long workout.

Stay hydrated: Proper hydration is essential during pregnancy, especially if you're experiencing nausea. Sip water before, during, and after your workouts to stay hydrated. Avoid exercising in hot and humid environments to prevent overheating.

Eat small, frequent meals: Nausea is a common symptom during the first trimester. To manage it, try eating small, frequent meals that are easy on your stomach. Choose nutritious foods that provide a steady source of energy, such as whole grains, lean proteins, fruits, and vegetables.

Practice relaxation techniques: Incorporate relaxation techniques into your routine to alleviate stress and promote a sense of calm. Deep breathing exercises, meditation, and gentle stretching can help you relax and reduce nausea and fatigue.

Get sufficient rest: Fatigue is a typical symptom during the first trimester. Choose sleep over everything and ensure you're getting enough rest each night. Listen to your body and allow yourself to take naps or rest when needed.

Consult your healthcare provider: Every pregnancy is unique, and it's crucial to consult your healthcare provider before making any significant changes to your fitness routine. They can provide personalized advice based on your health and guide you on what exercises are safe for you and your baby.

Remember, the first trimester is a time of significant changes in your body, and it's essential to be gentle and patient with yourself. Adapt your fitness routine to suit your needs and prioritize your well-being. By making mindful choices and staying in tune with your body, you can navigate nausea and fatigue while maintaining a healthy and active pregnancy.

Second trimester: modifying for growing belly

Congratulations on reaching your second trimester of pregnancy! This period brings exciting changes, including the visible growth of your belly. As you progress through this stage, it's essential to modify and adapt your fitness routine to accommodate your changing body. Here are some tips to help you maintain a safe and effective fitness routine during the second trimester while accommodating your growing belly:

Consult with your healthcare provider: Before making any modifications to your fitness routine, it's crucial to consult with your healthcare provider. They can provide personalized guidance based on your health, previous exercise habits, and any pregnancy-related factors.

Choose low-impact exercises: As your belly grows, opting for low-impact exercises can help reduce the strain on your joints and minimize the risk of injury. Activities such as walking, swimming, stationary cycling, and prenatal yoga are excellent options to consider.

Modify abdominal exercises: Traditional abdominal exercises like crunches and sit-ups should be avoided or modified during the second trimester. As your belly expands, these exercises can strain your abdominal muscles and potentially harm your baby. Instead, focus on exercises that engage your deep core muscles, such as pelvic tilts and modified planks, which can help maintain core strength.

Support your changing body: As your belly grows, your center of gravity shifts, which may affect your balance. Ensure you have proper support and stability during your workouts. Wear supportive footwear, avoid sudden movements, and consider using stability aids, such as a stability ball or a chair, to provide balance while exercising.

Stay hydrated and avoid overheating: Pregnancy increases your body's temperature, so it's important to stay hydrated during your workouts. Drinking plenty of water before, during, and after exercising is very important. Additionally, avoid exercising in hot and humid environments to prevent overheating, which can be harmful to both you and your baby.

Listen to your body: Pay close attention to how your body feels during exercise. If you experience any discomfort, pain, dizziness, or shortness of breath, stop exercising immediately and consult your healthcare provider. Your body is going through significant changes, and it's important to respect its signals.

Incorporate pelvic floor exercises: Strengthening your pelvic floor muscles can be beneficial during pregnancy and aid in postpartum recovery. Consider incorporating Kegel exercises into your fitness routine. These exercises involve contracting and relaxing the muscles that support your bladder, uterus, and bowels. Consult with your healthcare provider to ensure you're performing them correctly.

third trimester: preparing for labor and delivery

Congratulations on entering the third trimester of your pregnancy! This is an exciting time as you approach the final stretch before meeting your little one. In the third trimester, it's important to focus on preparing for labour and delivery. Here are some important points to note down :

Prenatal Care: Don't stop attending regular prenatal check-ups with your healthcare provider. They will monitor your health and the baby's growth, as well as address any concerns or questions you may have. These appointments are crucial for ensuring a healthy pregnancy.

Childbirth Education: Consider enrolling in childbirth education classes. These classes provide valuable information about the labor and delivery process, breathing techniques, pain management options, and what to expect during each stage of childbirth. They can help you feel more prepared and confident as the due date approaches.

Birth Plan: Discuss your birth preferences with your healthcare provider and create a birth plan. A birth plan outlines your preferences for pain management, positions during labor, who will be present in the delivery room, and any special requests you may have. Keep in mind that flexibility is essential as labor and delivery can be unpredictable.

Physical Preparation: Stay active and engage in regular exercise, unless advised otherwise by your healthcare provider. Prenatal yoga, swimming, walking, and gentle stretching can help maintain strength and flexibility, which can be beneficial during labor. However, listen to your body and avoid any activities that cause discomfort or pain.

Emotional Well-being: Take time to nurture your emotional well-being during this phase. Surround yourself with a supportive network of family and friends, attend prenatal support groups, and communicate openly with your partner or a trusted confidant. It's normal to have a range of emotions, including excitement, anxiety, and fear . Don't forget to take care of yourself and seek professional help if needed.

Nesting and Preparing the Home: Use this time to prepare your home for the arrival of your baby. Set up the nursery, wash and organize baby clothes, and gather essential items such as diapers, blankets, and feeding supplies. Creating a nurturing and comfortable environment can help you feel more ready for your baby's arrival.

Pack Your Hospital Bag: Start packing your hospital bag with essential items you'll need during your stay. Include comfortable clothing, toiletries, nursing bras, baby outfits, and any other personal items that will make you feel more at ease during the hospital stay. Check with your healthcare provider or hospital for a comprehensive list of recommended items.

Birth Partner's Role: Discuss the role of your birth partner, whether it's your partner, a family member, or a doula. Talk about their involvement during labor, their support strategies, and any specific tasks they should be aware of. This will ensure that you both have a clear understanding of each other's expectations.

Remember, every pregnancy and birth experience is unique. Do not feel reluctant to reach out to your healthcare provider with any questions or concerns you may have. Trust in your body's ability to bring new life into the world, and embrace this transformative journey.

Wishing you a safe and smooth delivery!

CHAPTER 7:

Special considerations for high-risk pregnancies

Gestational diabetes and exercise

Gestational diabetes mellitus (GDM) is a condition characterized by high blood sugar levels that develop during pregnancy. It affects approximately 2-10% of pregnant women worldwide. Proper management of gestational diabetes is crucial to promote maternal and fetal health. One aspect of management includes incorporating regular exercise into the pregnancy routine. In this note, we will explore the benefits of exercise during pregnancy for women with gestational diabetes and provide some guidelines for safe and effective exercise.

Benefits of Exercise during Pregnancy for Gestational Diabetes:

Blood sugar regulation: Regular physical activity helps improve insulin sensitivity, allowing the body to use glucose more efficiently. This can help regulate blood sugar levels and reduce the risk of complications associated with gestational diabetes.

Weight management: Exercise plays a key role in maintaining a healthy weight during pregnancy. It helps control excessive weight gain, which is a risk factor for developing gestational diabetes and other pregnancy-related complications.

Cardiovascular health: Pregnancy increases the workload on the heart and circulatory system. Engaging in aerobic exercises like walking, swimming, or cycling can improve cardiovascular fitness, enhance circulation, and lower the risk of developing hypertension and preeclampsia.

Mood and well-being: Pregnancy can bring about hormonal changes and emotional challenges. Regular exercise releases endorphins, which can alleviate stress, improve mood, and boost overall well-being.

Guidelines for Exercise during Pregnancy with Gestational Diabetes:

Consult your healthcare provider: Before starting an exercise program, consult your healthcare provider or obstetrician. They will evaluate your individual circumstances, medical history, and assess any potential risks or contraindications.

Choose low-impact activities: Opt for low-impact exercises that are gentle on the joints, such as walking, swimming, prenatal yoga, or stationary cycling. These activities minimize the risk of injury and provide cardiovascular benefits.

Stay hydrated: Drink plenty of water before, during, and after exercises to stay hydrated so that you can prevent overheating. Avoid exercising when the environment is hot and humid .

Pace yourself: Gradually increase the duration and intensity of your exercise sessions over time. Start with shorter sessions and low-intensity exercises, then gradually progress as your body adapts.

Monitor blood sugar levels: Check your blood sugar levels before, during, and after exercise to ensure they remain within the target range. If levels are too low or too high, adjust your exercise routine or consult your healthcare provider for further guidance.

Listen to your body: Pay attention to any warning signs or discomfort during exercise, such as dizziness, shortness of breath, chest pain, or vaginal bleeding. If you experience any of these symptoms, stop exercising and seek medical advice.

Exercise is an essential component of managing gestational diabetes during pregnancy. It offers numerous benefits, including improved blood sugar regulation, weight management, cardiovascular health, and overall well-being. However, it is crucial to consult with your healthcare provider and follow safe guidelines to ensure a healthy and enjoyable exercise routine throughout your pregnancy.

Preeclampsia and hypertension management

Pregnancy is a critical period in a woman's life that requires special attention to her health and well-being. Preeclampsia and hypertension are two conditions that can potentially pose risks to both the mother and the developing fetus. Proper management of these conditions is crucial to ensure a safe and healthy pregnancy. Additionally, exercise during pregnancy, when done correctly and under medical supervision, can provide numerous benefits for both the mother and the baby. This note aims to provide an overview of preeclampsia and hypertension management, as well as the role of exercise during pregnancy.

Preeclampsia and Hypertension Management:

Regular prenatal care: Early and regular prenatal visits are essential to monitor blood pressure, detect any signs of preeclampsia, and manage hypertension effectively. Prenatal care involves regular check-ups, blood pressure monitoring, and urine tests to assess protein levels.

Blood pressure control: Blood pressure control is a key aspect of managing hypertension during pregnancy. Lifestyle modifications such as maintaining a healthy diet, reducing sodium intake, and avoiding excessive weight gain are important. Sometimes, medications will be prescribed to manage hypertension.

Monitoring for preeclampsia symptoms:
Preeclampsia is characterized by high blood pressure
and the presence of protein in the urine after 20 weeks
of pregnancy. Regular monitoring of symptoms such as
persistent headaches, blurred vision, sudden weight
gain, and swelling in the hands and face is crucial. Any
signs of preeclampsia should be reported to a
healthcare provider immediately.

Bed rest and activity modification: In some cases of
severe preeclampsia or hypertension, healthcare
providers may recommend bed rest or modified activity
levels to reduce stress and improve blood pressure
control. However, the exact recommendations should be
discussed with a healthcare provider as individual
circumstances may vary.

Exercise During Pregnancy:

Consultation with a healthcare provider: Before
starting or continuing an exercise regimen during
pregnancy, it is essential to consult with a healthcare
provider. They can assess the individual's health,
consider any complications or risks, and provide
personalized recommendations.

Benefits of exercise: Regular exercise during
pregnancy, when done appropriately, can provide
several benefits. It helps maintain a healthy weight,

improves mood, boosts energy levels, promotes better sleep, and enhances overall cardiovascular health.

Safe exercises during pregnancy: Low-impact exercises such as walking, swimming, stationary cycling, and prenatal yoga are generally considered safe during pregnancy. These exercises help maintain fitness levels without putting excessive strain on the joints or abdominal muscles.

Precautions and guidelines: Pregnant women should avoid activities that involve a high risk of falling, such as contact sports or vigorous activities with a high impact on the joints. It is important to listen to the body, avoid overexertion, and stay adequately hydrated during exercise.

Warning signs to stop exercising: While exercise during pregnancy is generally safe, it is crucial to be aware of warning signs that indicate a need to stop exercising. These include vaginal bleeding, dizziness or faintness, chest pain, shortness of breath, severe headache, and muscle weakness. If any of these symptoms occur, seek for immediate medical attention.

Preeclampsia and hypertension management during pregnancy require regular prenatal care, blood pressure control, and close monitoring for symptoms. Exercise, when done appropriately and under medical guidance, can provide numerous benefits during pregnancy. However, it is essential to consult with a healthcare provider, follow safety guidelines, and take good care of yourself.

Multiple pregnancies and exercise modifications

When it comes to multiple pregnancies, such as twins, triplets, or more, it is important to consider certain exercise modifications to ensure the safety and well-being of both the mother and the babies. Multiple pregnancies can place additional strain on the body, and exercising without proper modifications can increase the risk of complications. Therefore, it is essential to consult with a healthcare provider or a qualified prenatal exercise specialist before engaging in any exercise routine during a multiple pregnancy. They can provide personalized recommendations based on the specific circumstances of the pregnancy.

Here are some general guidelines and exercise modifications that may be recommended for women with multiple pregnancies:

Prioritize Safety: Safety should always be the top priority. Avoid activities with a high risk of falling or abdominal trauma, such as contact sports, horseback riding, skiing, or vigorous abdominal exercises.

Regular Check-ups: Maintain regular prenatal check-ups to monitor the progress of the pregnancy and ensure that there are no complications that might affect exercise recommendations.

Low-Impact Exercises: Choose low-impact exercises that are gentle on the joints and reduce the risk of injury. Walking, swimming, stationary cycling, and prenatal yoga are excellent choices for maintaining cardiovascular fitness and muscle strength without excessive strain.

Pelvic Floor Exercises: Engage in regular pelvic floor exercises, such as Kegels, to strengthen the pelvic floor muscles. This can help support the added weight and strain on the body during a multiple pregnancy and prepare for childbirth and postpartum recovery.

Core Strengthening: Focus on core-strengthening exercises that are safe for multiple pregnancies. Modified planks, pelvic tilts, and gentle abdominal exercises under the guidance of a qualified professional can help maintain core strength and stability.

Listen to Your Body: Pay attention to the signals your body gives and adjust the intensity and duration of exercise accordingly. As the pregnancy progresses, the body's capabilities may change, and modifications might be necessary. Fatigue, dizziness, shortness of breath, or any unusual discomfort should be taken as cues to slow down or stop exercising.

Adequate Rest and Recovery: Multiple pregnancies can be physically demanding, so make sure to prioritize rest and recovery. Get enough sleep and allow ample time for your body to recover between exercise sessions.

Remember, every multiple pregnancy is unique, and exercise recommendations may vary depending on factors such as the number of babies, maternal health, and any existing complications. Always consult with your healthcare provider before starting or modifying an exercise routine during a multiple pregnancy to ensure the safety of both the mother and the babies.

CHAPTER 8:

POSTPARTUM RECOVERY AND RETURNING TO FITNESS

Understanding the postpartum body

Congratulations on the arrival of your little one! As you embark on this beautiful journey of motherhood, I wanted to take a moment to discuss the postpartum body and offer some insights that may help you understand and embrace the changes that occur during this phase.

The postpartum period is a unique and transformative time for a woman's body. After nine months of carrying and nourishing a growing life, your body undergoes significant physical and hormonal changes as it recovers and adjusts to the new demands of motherhood. Understanding and accepting these changes can be empowering and instrumental in fostering a positive body image.

Physical changes: During pregnancy, your body undergoes various adaptations to accommodate your growing baby. It's natural to expect some physical changes postpartum. These may include a softer belly, stretched skin, and enlarged breasts due to milk production. Remember that these changes are temporary, and your body will gradually recover and regain its pre-pregnancy form.

Hormonal fluctuations: Hormones play a crucial role in pregnancy and childbirth, and they continue to fluctuate in the postpartum period. These hormonal shifts can contribute to mood swings, fatigue, and changes in your body's shape and size. Be patient with yourself as your body and hormones find their balance.

Healing process: Giving birth is a remarkable feat, and your body needs time to heal. Whether you had a vaginal delivery or a cesarean section, allow yourself ample time for recovery. Follow your healthcare provider's guidance on postpartum care, including rest, proper nutrition, gentle exercises, and any necessary medical interventions. Embrace self-care and prioritize your well-being as you navigate this healing journey.

Embracing your new body: Your postpartum body may look different from what you were accustomed to, and that's perfectly normal. Embrace the changes and appreciate the incredible strength and resilience your body has shown throughout pregnancy and childbirth. Focus on the joy and love your baby brings rather than getting caught up in societal expectations of postpartum body ideals.

Seeking support: Remember that you are not alone on this journey. Reach out to your partner, family, or friends for emotional support. Join local or online communities of new moms who can provide understanding, advice, and encouragement. Connecting with other women who are experiencing or have experienced similar changes can be reassuring and empowering.

Lastly, be kind to yourself. Adjusting to your new role as a mother takes time, and it's essential to prioritize self-care and self-compassion. Celebrate the strength and beauty of your postpartum body, as it has accomplished something truly miraculous.

Wishing you a joyful and fulfilling postpartum journey.

Recovering from vaginal and cesarean births

Recovering from vaginal and cesarean births can be a unique and personal experience for each woman. Both types of childbirth involve physical changes and require adequate rest, self-care, and support to ensure a smooth recovery. Here are some general guidelines for recovering from vaginal and cesarean births:

Recovering from Vaginal Birth:

Rest and take it easy: After giving birth vaginally, it's essential to prioritize rest and allow your body time to heal. Get plenty of sleep, and avoid strenuous activities during the early weeks of recovery.

Manage pain and discomfort: It's normal to experience soreness, perineal discomfort, and swelling after a vaginal birth. Applying ice packs or warm compresses, using pain medication as prescribed by your healthcare provider, and practicing good perineal hygiene can help alleviate discomfort.

Care for your perineum: If you had an episiotomy or tearing during delivery, proper perineal care is crucial. Keep the area clean and dry, use a peri-bottle or warm water to cleanse after urination and bowel movements, and change sanitary pads frequently.

Practice pelvic floor exercises: Strengthening your pelvic floor muscles can aid in the recovery process. Perform Kegel exercises regularly to regain muscle tone and improve bladder control. Consult with your healthcare provider for guidance on proper technique.

Take care of your emotional well-being: Adjusting to life with a newborn can be overwhelming, so it's essential to prioritize self-care. Let your partner, family, or friends support you , and consider joining a postpartum support group to connect with other new mothers.

Recovering from Caesarean Birth (C-Section):

Allow your body to heal: Recovering from a caesarean birth involves healing from both childbirth and surgery. Take it easy, and avoid lifting heavy things or strenuous activities. Follow your healthcare provider's instructions on how to care for your incision and when to remove dressings.

Manage pain and discomfort: Pain and discomfort around the incision area are common after a C-section. Take pain medication as prescribed by your healthcare provider, and use supportive measures such as applying ice packs or using a heating pad (if approved by your doctor) to relieve discomfort.

Monitor your incision: Keep a close eye on your incision site for signs of infection, such as redness, swelling, or discharge. Report any concerns to your healthcare provider promptly.

Gradually increase physical activity: While it's important to rest initially, engaging in gentle movements and light exercises can promote circulation and aid in recovery. Start with short walks and gradually increase your activity level as advised by your healthcare provider.

Seek emotional support: Recovering from a C-section can sometimes bring emotional challenges. Reach out to your loved ones or a mental health professional if you're feeling overwhelmed or struggling with your emotions.

Remember that every woman's recovery journey is different, and it's essential to consult with your healthcare provider for personalized guidance. They can provide specific recommendations based on your unique circumstances and address any concerns you may have.

Safe and effective postpartum exercise guidelines

Congratulations on the arrival of your baby! As you embark on your postpartum journey, it's important to prioritize your physical well-being while gradually easing back into exercise. Here are some guidelines to ensure safe and effective postpartum exercise:

Consult with your healthcare provider: Before starting any postpartum exercise routine, consult your healthcare provider to ensure you have received clearance to engage in physical activity. They can provide personalized recommendations based on your specific health needs and recovery progress.

Start gradually: Your body has undergone significant changes during pregnancy and childbirth, so it's essential to start slowly and gradually increase the intensity and duration of your workouts. Begin with gentle exercises, such as walking or pelvic floor exercises, and listen to your body's cues.

Focus on core and pelvic floor exercises: The core and pelvic floor muscles play a crucial role during pregnancy and childbirth. Engaging in exercises that target these muscles can help strengthen and restore their function. Examples include pelvic tilts, kegels, and deep abdominal exercises like diaphragmatic breathing.

Pay attention to posture: Poor posture can be common after childbirth due to increased strain on the back and neck. Be mindful of your posture during exercises and throughout the day. Maintain proper alignment by keeping your shoulders relaxed, spine neutral, and core engaged.

Include cardiovascular exercises: Gradually incorporate cardiovascular exercises into your routine to improve cardiovascular fitness and overall endurance. Activities like brisk walking, swimming, or low-impact aerobics are gentle on the joints and can be easily modified to match your fitness level.

Prioritize rest and recovery: Your body needs time to heal and recover after childbirth. Allow yourself ample rest and listen to your body's signals. Don't push yourself too hard and ensure you're getting sufficient sleep and nutrition to support your postpartum recovery.

Be mindful of breastfeeding considerations: If you're breastfeeding, it's important to consider its impact on exercise. Plan your workouts around nursing sessions to avoid discomfort and potential milk supply issues. Supportive sports bras and nursing pads can provide added comfort and protection during exercise.

Stay hydrated and nourished: It's important to drink plenty of water before, during, and after your workouts to stay hydrated. Also, ensure you're consuming a balanced diet that includes nutrient-dense foods to support your energy levels and overall health.

Seek professional guidance if needed: If you're unsure about the right exercises or technique, consider seeking guidance from a qualified postnatal fitness professional or physical therapist. They can provide expert advice tailored to your specific needs and help you develop a safe and effective exercise plan.

Remember, every woman's postpartum journey is unique, and it's crucial to listen to your body and give yourself time to heal. By following these guidelines, you can gradually regain your strength and fitness while prioritizing your well-being. Enjoy the process and celebrate each small step forward!

Building a support system and finding balance

The postpartum period can be a beautiful yet challenging time for new mothers. As you navigate the joys and demands of motherhood, it's crucial to build a strong support system and find a balance that works for you. Here are some important points to write down :

Reach out to loved ones: Don't hesitate to lean on your family and friends for support during this time. They can help with household chores, meal preparation, or even taking care of the baby while you rest. Accepting help from others is not a sign of weakness but rather a way to ensure you have the time and energy to focus on your own well-being.

Seek professional help: Consider engaging the services of healthcare professionals, such as a lactation consultant, postpartum doula, or a therapist specializing in maternal mental health. These experts can provide guidance, education, and emotional support tailored to your specific needs. Always know that asking for help signifies strength and self-care .

Join a support group: Connecting with other new mothers who are going through similar experiences can be immensely beneficial. Look for local or online support groups where you can share your thoughts, concerns, and joys with people who understand what you're going through. These groups can provide validation, advice, and lasting friendships.

Prioritize self-care: Amidst the demands of caring for a newborn, it's vital to prioritize your own well-being. Self-care can take various forms, such as taking short breaks, practicing relaxation techniques like deep breathing or meditation, engaging in activities you enjoy, or simply getting enough sleep. Remember that by taking care of yourself, you're better able to care for your baby.

Establish boundaries: Communicate your needs and set boundaries with your loved ones. It's important to have open and honest conversations about what you require during this time. Setting boundaries will help you manage your time, energy, and emotions effectively, ensuring that you're able to give your best to both your baby and yourself.

Embrace flexibility: Adjusting to the demands of motherhood can be overwhelming, and it's normal to feel like you're constantly juggling responsibilities. Remember that it's okay to let go of perfection and embrace flexibility. Adapt to the needs of your baby and yourself, and be kind to yourself during this transition period.

Stay connected: Maintain social connections with friends and engage in activities outside of motherhood. Carving out time for yourself and nurturing relationships beyond your role as a mother will help you maintain a sense of identity and fulfillment.

Building a support system and finding balance after giving birth is a process that takes time and patience. Be gentle with yourself, celebrate your successes, and seek help when needed. Remember, you are not alone, and there are resources and people available to support you on this incredible journey of motherhood.

CONCLUSION:

EMPOWERING YOURSELF ON THE JOURNEY TO MOTHERHOOD

In the book titled "PREGNANT BUT FIT " we have explored the transformative journey of pregnancy and the significance of empowering oneself during this special time. Pregnancy is a remarkable experience that brings joy, anticipation, and sometimes challenges. It is crucial for expectant mothers to prioritize their physical and emotional well-being, as it not only benefits them but also contributes to the healthy development of their unborn child.

Throughout this book, we have emphasized the importance of maintaining a balanced and active lifestyle during pregnancy. The workouts and exercises provided have been carefully tailored to meet the unique needs of pregnant women, focusing on safety, strength, flexibility, and overall fitness. By engaging in regular physical activity, women can enhance their endurance, improve their posture, and manage discomfort that may arise during pregnancy.

However, empowerment during pregnancy extends far beyond physical fitness. It involves cultivating a positive mindset, building a strong support system, and making informed choices about one's healthcare. As an expectant mother, it is crucial to become an active participant in your prenatal care, engaging in open and honest conversations with your healthcare provider, and seeking guidance when needed.

The journey to motherhood can sometimes be overwhelming, filled with various emotions and uncertainties. It is essential for women to nurture their emotional well-being during this time. Self-care practices such as meditation, relaxation techniques, and seeking emotional support from loved ones can greatly contribute to a sense of calm and balance.

Empowerment also entails being knowledgeable about the changes occurring in your body and understanding the needs of your growing baby. Educating yourself about pregnancy, childbirth, and postpartum care equips you with the confidence to make informed decisions and actively participate in the birthing process.

Remember, every woman's journey to motherhood is unique, and it is important to honour and celebrate that individuality. Embrace the changes your body undergoes, cherish the bond you form with your baby, and surround yourself with positivity and love. The journey may have its ups and downs, but with empowerment, you can navigate the challenges with strength and grace.

As you embark on this beautiful chapter of your life, I encourage you to embrace the lessons shared in this book and continue to empower yourself on the journey to motherhood. By prioritizing your physical and emotional well-being, seeking knowledge, and nurturing a supportive environment, you are not only benefiting yourself but also creating a strong foundation for your little miracle to thrive. Congratulations on this incredible journey, and may it be filled with joy, love, and empowerment.